T0208886

How to Get the Perfect Brazilian Wax

A Step-By-Step Guide to Getting the Perfect Brazilian and Finding Your Inner Goddess

Molly Aldrich

iUniverse, Inc.
New York   Bloomington

How to Get the Perfect Brazilian Wax
A Step-By-Step Guide to Getting the Perfect Brazilian and Finding Your Inner Goddess

The views expressed in this work are solely those of the author and do not necessarily reflect the views of the publisher, and the publisher hereby disclaims any responsibility for them.

iUniverse books may be ordered through booksellers or by contacting:

iUniverse
1663 Liberty Drive
Bloomington, IN 47403
www.iuniverse.com
1-800-Authors (1-800-288-4677)

Because of the dynamic nature of the Internet, any Web addresses or links contained in this book may have changed since publication and may no longer be valid. The views expressed in this work are solely those of the author and do not necessarily reflect the views of the publisher, and the publisher hereby disclaims any responsibility for them.

ISBN: 978-1-4401-2419-8 (pbk)
ISBN: 978-1-4401-2420-4 (ebk)

Library of Congress Control Number: 2009922644

Printed in the United States of America

iUniverse rev. date: 2/12/2009

Dedication

To my father, who taught me that sensitivity and compassion are a measure of one's intelligence. To my mom, for raising three independent girls with love, kindness, and spirituality. They worked together to keep me grounded and open to the mystery of the universe. To my two older sisters, who taught me everything about becoming a woman and loving myself. To my "harem" of girlfriends. To the men who love women. To all the beautiful goddesses whom I have been fortunate to meet in my life. Every one of you has inspired my own journey of self-healing and awareness. I am so fortunate and blessed.... My deepest gratitude to all of you.

Contents

Foreword

I wrote this book as an instruction manual so that everyone could understand the mysterious process of getting a Brazilian wax. I have also included testimonials throughout the book, from women of every age, background, and lifestyle. Some of my testimonials chose to use different names or exclude certain personal facts, but each testimonial is honest and real. There are funny parts and graphic parts to this manual. I have a very honest and down to earth personality. But the reason I included "Finding Your Inner Goddess", as my subtitle is the real heart and soul of this book. Getting a "Brazilian" is a step toward recognizing your potential as a woman who is sexy and desirable—a goddess. I have come to learn, through giving Brazilians all these years that women don't talk enough with each other about what they really want to talk about! We want to understand our bodies and appreciate them. We want our partners to love and cherish them. It is amazing to me that every day, women, like the one quoted below, come in and unload their fears and insecurities about their sexuality, their bodies, and their vaginas.

> What? A Brazilian? Me? Certainly not two years ago. I had never even heard of such a thing. And now? I wouldn't think of missing my appointment! I'm a stay-at-home mom, on the curvy side, forty-nine years old, and there really is nothing outwardly sexy about me. So, why do I bother with getting a Brazilian? Let's state the obvious. My husband loves it. And I love that he loves it. But there's more to it than that. I have a secret. One that I don't need to share. A secret that is more powerful by being kept. There are, of course, the extra sensual

and sexual sensitivities that are brought forth by that clean skin experience. Yummy! And it's all mine.

Jane Plain, 49

There is no reason a woman should ever feel guilt about wanting to be beautiful and desired. That is who we are. We are women who feel intensely. We know the secrets of life, death, birth, and sex. We are the gatekeepers of all life, nurturing, and intuition. We are magnificent and perfect. Every woman on the planet deserves to feel her power as a goddess.

Brazilians are personal. I do this work so that women have the opportunity to recognize their inherent gift of the divine feminine. Our vaginas deserve this recognition, and, through them, we can find our true selves. Through our love for our own, we can help teach our daughters, sisters, and mothers to nurture and love themselves. Their health and our health depend on our acknowledgment. We are the template for all creation!

I consider Brazilian waxing to be goddess work. I love, respect, admire, adore, and feel completely comfortable working with and touching this most sacred area of women. My ultimate goal with every woman when she enters the room is that she leaves feeling completely sexy and confident. This will help her to become more in touch with her own body and sexuality. I consider every person who enters my room a guest, and it is an honor to have them in my space. A space where one can feel free and safe to ask questions or experience finding themselves. I have had many guests in my sanctuary of pussy love who honestly just want to feel clean "down there"; however, they have no interest in seeing their sacred spot and never have. At those moments, I feel like Brazilians are a path to self-love and goddess healing that everyone deserves to experience. That is why I felt inspired to write this manual and why love what I do!

My name is Tricia, and I am a forty-two-year-old engineer, so, by nature, fairly conservative. Before I turned forty, I decided that I needed to step out of my self-imposed box and mark the occasion by doing something spectacular for myself to celebrate this next phase of my life. After a great deal of thought and self-reflection, I saw this advertisement for a photography studio that specialized in black-and-white nude photography. *This, I thought, sounds like the perfect way to celebrate finally being comfortable in my own skin and feeling like a beautiful woman.* I met with the photographer, and he had many nuggets of advice to prepare for our session, including having a Brazilian wax. He said that the hair would detract from the grace and beauty of the body lines, and, although I could shave, he wouldn't recommend it. So, I randomly called Molly and nervously set my first appointment. Going in for the wax appointment, I didn't know what to expect, so I explained to Molly that I was a waxing "virgin" and why I was getting it done. She was so upbeat and supportive that I eventually relaxed and trusted her to proceed. She assured me that I would become addicted to waxes. At the time, and even after that first wax experience, I wasn't sure that I believed her, but once I got those photos back and I saw how incredible my body looked in those photos, I was convinced! I am now addicted to Brazilian waxes, as Molly had predicted and, even though the look is part of it, each wax is actually a small celebration of this more contented phase of my life and a reminder that I really do love this body.

Tricia, 42, engineer

Chapter 1
Why Get a Brazilian?

So why get a Brazilian? There are several levels of reasoning beyond what I mentioned in the foreword, but let's discuss the most obvious. Getting a Brazilian wax will make you feel cleaner down there and improve your sex life. A Brazilian is a fun way to ignite your romantic life and feel sexy. It can be seen as simple as that, however I feel Brazilian's can be viewed on a deeper level. We fix our hair, get pedicures, and wear lipstick and nice clothes to create a desire from our partners or even just to feel good about ourselves. These acts of grooming attract a mate, but when this mate reaches your sweet spot, you have ignored the very purpose of your hard work! You cook dinner and prepare a nice home environment to show your love, so that you may be appreciated and desired. But you exclude preparing your very source of power. We work hard to be successful so that we feel better about ourselves, yet ignore the very purpose of our existence … the holy spot that holds all the creation and mystery of our universe.

Have you ever experienced for yourself or watched another person lose weight? It is amazing to watch this transformation; I have experienced this firsthand. Once the weight starts to melt off, you begin to want to fix your hair more, you desire to get new clothes, you begin to feel good about yourself, and you accept that you are safe to finally be seen.

> I had been married for a long time and was suddenly faced with a divorce I wasn't exactly ready for. A friend of mine suggested some pampering, a facial, and perhaps an eyebrow wax. The esthetician suggested a bikini wax, and my friend applied the pressure to follow through.

I have to say I was shy and a little embarrassed to be lying on the table with my legs up in the air with a complete stranger. Something that hadn't happened in my world for over ten years. It hurt. I was done.

But I felt different. I felt sexy. I went back and got a pedicure and a manicure and waxed again. I found Molly, whom I love, and made a standing appointment. I began dating again although I waited the "morally appropriate" time to begin sleeping with my boyfriend; I did so with a passion and personal abandonment my husband never saw. I'll never go back. It is part of my grooming habits now.

Sue, 41, PhD in education and human resource studies/ educator

Getting a Brazilian is one of those steps you can take that will inspire you to do even more for yourself. This is not just about attracting a partner or pleasing another. Brazilians are a tool in the toolbox of life, which allows a woman to declare to herself that she is sensual and sexy—a hot goddess. It is about stepping into the light, and the recognition of ourselves through our vaginas.

My first Brazilian was a wedding gift for my husband. The subsequent waxings really have nothing to do with him, although he doesn't complain. There is something empowering and liberating about having a Brazilian waxing done. It gives me a feeling of being in charge of my body and creates a feeling of inward sexiness that otherwise doesn't exist.

Jenny, 42, teacher/flower grower

It's not just the Brazilian wax itself that holds the key, but the recognition and attention to our bodies that is so vital in our world. Begin to acknowledge the existence of our perfection through using The Law of Attraction. Use The Law of Attraction, by performing physical and mindful awareness. This physical and mindful awareness will draw the love and attention to our bodies and vagina's that one deserves. In using The Law of Attraction one can take a physical step or perform a ritual to help guide us to ultimately realizing how beautiful and sacred our vaginas are.... Every society in the world performs rituals to help them connect with a higher purpose. We practice these rituals to remind us of the importance of something that has a higher purpose. Ritual is such a beautiful practice, which is often overlooked in our culture. We practice some rituals every day unconsciously, like brushing our teeth, in order to work toward something bigger in our lives, like keeping our teeth healthy! We must sometimes take these little steps and perform these rituals in order to step into the light of transformation and knowledge. If you practice anything enough, it will become habit. Practice the steps and perform the ritual of embracing your sexuality through the ancient art of waxing.

The Western culture is just beginning to explore the link between one's spiritual and sexual selves. Many cultures practice the ancient teachings of the female Taoist, which influenced the Japanese geisha and Chinese white tigress. These teachings all express the importance of waxing as one of the ways to embrace one's sexual energy. Sexual energy is the reason we are born and it is the reason we age and die. Sexual energy is about procreation, recreation, and transformation. Through the ancient practice of waxing you will begin to see yourself as I see you and as the universe has recognized you ... *as a woman!*

> This may sound insane to many of you, but it took a long time for me to finally give up on my marriage even after finding out my husband was involved in homosexual activity while we were married. With two young daughters, a demanding career in surgery, and a strong desire to not pass on a heritage of divorce to my children, I hung in there like a pit bull, hoping somehow that we could manage to heal our marriage and my broken heart, if my husband agreed to stay faithful to me. What I didn't realize is how untrue I was being to that much wounded heart. I had buried my femininity, sexuality, and trust somewhere deep inside for safe keeping, far away from my husband and even myself. I was a mom, a surgeon, and a life partner. I was blessed to have what I had. I was trying to make it work somehow. Finally, I realized I just couldn't do it anymore. I was deeply unhappy and frightened that it was only

a matter of time before he acted out again. The most painful day was that day I realized I was being unfaithful to me.

So began the painful process of divorce and rediscovering myself. I needed something to remind me of who I was as a woman, a celebration of my femininity and, to some extent, a proclamation of my sexuality. Some women change how they dress or buy a new car or change their hair color to proclaim their independence and their new selves after divorce. I needed to do something no else could see but me. The Brazilian symbolized the new me: a feminine, sexual, beautiful creature, a bearer of the image of God, who formed us exactly as He intended. It was to reveal to anyone in the future who would see me unclothed and completely available to be explored and touched: "I am to be cherished. I have no secrets. I am female to the core. Love me for who I am."

Sherri, 42, surgeon

Chapter 2
I'm the Brazilian Waxing Master

So what makes me the "Brazilian Waxing Master"? I will tell you all my credentials because I know there are different women reading this, and some of them need intellectual reasons to believe what I say. Hopefully, by the end of this manual, along with the other half of the readers, they will connect with the spiritual, beaver-loving, pussy-fanatic vagina worshippers out there who find themselves loving the Brazilian for the way it makes them feel in the head, heart, soul, and body!

I have been waxing for about fifteen years, professionally for about ten years, with an esthetician license. Once I got my license, I was very lucky to be hired by a major salon immediately after graduation. I was very good at what I did right away; I am one of those people who, once they have their minds on something, strive to be the very best. I waxed every friend, sister, mom, acquaintance, and stranger I could find. Every time I heard about a good waxer in town, I made an appointment with him or her and carefully examined every motion, tool, language, and position, plus the waxer's general demeanor—anything I could learn from. I went to three-day-long Brazilian waxing classes. I bought videos, read books, and researched on the Internet; you name it, and I have experienced it with a detective's eye. I had brave friends get on my table with legs wide open while I stretched one vagina lip in one direction and asked what that felt like. I have pulled butt cheeks apart and discovered which position made them feel the most comfortable and which got the most hair! I have explored, pulled, opened, stretched, researched, experimented, and asked a million questions to earn this title of Master Waxer.

I wax a minimum of fifteen crotches a day, and during spring break I don't even know … but you figure a ten-hour day, and my waxes are fifteen-minute appointments … wow, it even makes me feel crazy to think about it right now in my little office far away from work! This also should make you realize, as I already know, that there are thousands of normal-looking women out there with a little secret in their panties! That serious-looking librarian, doctor, scientist, teacher, housewife, or clerk that you would never expect to, might be a goddess in disguise! I have seen every sort of woman you can imagine come into my room. I have witnessed transformations of self-love and appreciation that make me feel amazing. I have experienced timid housewives who come back with tales of finding the secret porn star within them. It has been the most enlightening journey of my life to share this opportunity of healing with women.

I must admit I was apprehensive about getting a Brazilian Wax for the first time. This fear wasn't only because of the expected pain and embarrassment, but I wondered what Molly would think of a woman in her fifties doing something like this. I always had the impression this kind of thing was only for young women. However, I've been getting a Brazilian wax for a couple of years now, and I love it! My husband couldn't be happier, and it sure adds some spice to our sex life. When it's time for a "waxing," he insists I call Molly and tell her I need to come in right away because it's a romantic emergency!

My original fear about getting a Brazilian Wax vanished as soon as I met Molly. She is a well-trained professional who makes me feel comfortable and normal while she artistically completes her work. I have also found that the pain associated with this process is overrated, and after a few times, it gets easier and easier. I'd recommend a Brazilian Wax to any woman who wants to feel and look sexy. I've also found it really doesn't matter if you are young in age but only that you are young at heart.

Jane, 56, works for the city

I am very difficult to get into, and most guests must prebook their appointments to make sure they will be able to get in several weeks later. There is one experience in particular that stands out to me, when I really started to realize that I might be a master. You must realize that, with people like me, who have to be the best at what they do, one of their worst or best qualities (however you view it) is that *no one* is harder on them than themselves. It is next to impossible to get me to believe that there isn't more to learn or a way I can do something better. So this moment made me have to step back and try to see in myself the possibility of my greatness and potential. It still feels weird to say, but I am trying to accept my gifts and skills and accept myself. So a guest from LA came in for a Brazilian wax, and I could tell immediately that she was a pretty fancy lady, but also very hard to please, or just that she had been around and had experienced some of the finest things in life, including waxing and spa treatments. At this point in the game, to be honest, no one made me nervous. I had been doing this long enough that I felt a little sense of expertise. So I treated her like every other guest out there. After the wax, she told me it was the best wax she had ever had! Okay, I have heard that before, but then she went on to explain that she has been getting waxed for years by the same woman in LA who waxes all the stars! So she did name-drop, but although I'm good at waxing, I don't know how it works and what kind of okays I need to drop names in a book. But let me tell you, the few names she dropped were fun ones, and the waxer's name is also very well known in my little underground industry. Here I am telling the story, years later, and my heart still races with the excitement and knowledge that I could be, or maybe am, a Master Waxer! Is this what it feels like to receive the greatest compliment of your life? It was for me!

I know we're all looking for something to be good at, something to validate our existence—a footprint, some recognition, that moment of knowing you're needed, or something! This waxing stuff is my passion and purpose. I have nurtured and fed my art of pussy! I am the Brazilian Waxing Master!

For years, I pondered how ladies of erotica achieved that sleek, bare look of their most intimate parts. I secretly wondered how I might feel or what I would look like, but always assumed it would involve a regimen of awkward and painful shaving, and naturally, I steered clear. Then a respected, and I might add, a very conservative friend told me she had been getting Brazilian waxes for years and loved them. It was quick, easy, and she had the very best person to do them, Molly. Well, my friend was right. After meeting Molly and getting my courage up, I, too, got my first Brazilian wax and think I may be hooked. I'm not quite sure if all my secret wonderings about feeling sleek and bare have been explored, but it's a start. Whether it's a woman's search for her own beauty, or sexiness, or connection to divine feminine, I'm glad the universe guided me to experience this new wonderment. I am thankful for the kind, gentle spirit Molly brings to her work and the safe, trusting place she creates to allow me to feel free.

Linda, 50, wife/stepmother/businesswoman

Chapter 3
What Is a Brazilian Wax?

So you want to know what a Brazilian wax is. That is the real reason you picked up this book, right? There are several different kinds of bikini waxes out there, and there are all kinds of names for them. I am going to give you the main industry names, so you know what to ask for, plus one of my personal and customer favorites that I invented.

Let us start with tamest and least amount of hair removed.

The Bikini Wax. This means the only hair that will be removed is the hair that sticks out of a standard swimsuit—that annoying hair that grows outside of the crease between your thigh/crotch and creeps down your leg! This may include a little off the top part of your natural bikini line if your hair grows up toward your belly button.

The Brazilian Wax. This wax leaves a vertical strip of hair starting a few inches above the lip and labia area going down the front of the vagina. So all the hair is removed from the sides, and, yes, ladies, the crack of your butt, including the perianal area. Some people choose to keep a one-finger width of a strip or a two-finger width. In a true Brazilian wax, the hair is not removed from the labia. However, most people do not know these technical terms, and if you make an appointment for a Brazilian, most waxers are prepared to remove the hair from the labia also.

The Playboy. This is actually a rather new name in the industry, which comes from the *Playboy* models in the famous magazine.

This is definitely the most popular and requested wax. The same hair is removed that takes place in the traditional Brazilian wax, but this time, the hair is also removed from the labia. So you are left with a thin strip of hair starting a few inches above the lip area that stops right above the lips, and the rest is clean, including the butt crack and perianal areas. You can still leave a thicker width of a vertical strip of hair, but the rest is smooth and hairless. In both the Brazilian and the playboy wax, hair growing up toward the belly button can also be removed.

The Sphinx. Again, if someone makes an appointment for a Brazilian wax, most waxers are prepared to also do the sphinx. In this wax, all the hair will be removed; all hair is removed from the labia, butt crack, and perianal area. You will be completely hairless and clean! Those of you who are Sex in the City fans might remember the joke of this particular wax being called the "Telly Savalas"—named after the famous bald actor!

The Extreme Bikini. This is my invention and is quickly becoming my most requested wax, and, because I want you to know everything, ladies … this is also the wax that I have! All the hair is removed from the sides but is taken in a few inches farther than the standard bikini wax. I keep the shape of a natural bikini line like a piece of pie. It's wider on the top but comes down at an angle right above the lips. The hair is removed from the labia, butt crack, and perianal area. Some ladies prefer to keep the hair on the labia, but everyone wants the butt crack done in my extreme bikini!

The Shape or The Design. You can request any shape or design. The most popular is a letter. I have done a lightning bolt, heart, moon, and Tiffany box! Be realistic about what shape would look good, and work with your waxer's suggestions for what would work on you. I have used color before, but this can be very challenging and time-consuming. Discuss this with your waxer before the appointment, if you want to do the shape or design wax.

I think I had better address that I love and appreciate a full bush of hair too! One of the reasons I maintain my own, leaving a little hair behind, is this theory: Boys waited their whole lives to get a glimpse of the ever-elusive pubic hair. They finally grew into men and finally got to see that hot hairy patch. So I do appreciate the visual of a natural, full woman. That is why my personal favorite is to leave a little hair behind for the visual aspect. But as you will discover in the coming chapters, it is so amazing to have that hair removed. And there is much to be said for appreciating and seeing yourself fully without that veil of hair hiding your beautiful self. No one is a bigger lover of the natural woman than I, but there is a reason that this ancient practice of waxing has stayed in every culture through the years. It is an opportunity to celebrate yourself and choose how you would like to look and feel.

Women are judged so much by their appearances; this was finally something about my appearance where only I could be the judge. Waxing made me feel so much better about myself; it's a very intimate experience. Being comfortable with your esthetician also makes the experience worthwhile.

Brielle, 27, construction project coordinator

I'm an advocate for finding your inner goddess and feeling sexy. So give yourself the gift of trying the different options, and discover which one makes you feel the most beautiful. If it's the full bush in all its glory, I support your choice, but try one of these just once!

My really nervous and shy guests usually like to start with the standard bikini wax and work themselves up to the sphinx. There are also those brave folks who have never even had their eyebrows waxed before but have decided they want to start with the sphinx and are then really happy they just got their first wax out of the way! I suggest that if you are truly interested in having a Brazilian or sphinx, you should just bite the bullet and get it done.

"Go Brazilian or Go Home." As a mother of three—what a way to re-energize your body and marriage. I have always been the conservative "bikini waxer." Just on the sides, maybe one extra strip, but not too much. Once I relaxed and let go, I was thrilled with the results (my husband was fired up too). Thank you for introducing me to this wonderful procedure. Brazilian all the way!

Staley,(age not included) mother

Chapter 4
Which Wax Is Best for You?

Now let's discuss some other factors that I consider before making the decision of which type of wax job is best for my guest. Most people want my opinion on what I think they should get, or they are just so nervous that they can't decide or can't picture which wax they would most like on themselves.

I consider the hair type—is it extremely coarse or on the softer side? If your hair type is extremely thick and coarse, you might want to think about the extreme bikini or the Brazilian with a thicker width of a strip. The reason a true Brazilian leaves that landing strip is because the hair that grows directly above the lip area is the most aggressive hair to remove. This strip of hair is also the hair that seems to grow back the quickest, in my experience, and seems to always be a little rough. My really die-hard guests with this coarser hair, over time of consistent waxing, who want to be good candidates for a sphinx, do eventually get the hair to soften up. So if your hair type is extremely coarse and thick consider keeping the strip, but if you want that smooth, clean sphinx, you will have to be a very consistent waxer and understand that it will be a process over time, to get that strip area working in your favor. But it will be well worth the commitment.

On the other side of the coin, if your hair is very light in color or texture, you might want to consider going with the sphinx. If your hair can't represent itself in an eye-appealing way with the strip left behind, then it can look a little silly. For example, if you only have few sparse curly hairs in the center strip or are a little patchy with a bald spot in that area, there is nothing to really hold the shape of a strip.

Now, let us think about the color of the hair in a little more detail. The obvious candidate for a sphinx is one who is going gray or turning white down there! Believe it or not, half of my guests are ladies in their forties, fifties, and sixties, who would rather see no hair down there than see it going gray. I hear this complaint so often, and I suggest the sphinx, and they return glowing, feeling sexy down there again, with much approval from their significant others! If your hair is blonde or red but dense, then you can keep the strip, still looking attractive, but if it's sparse with these hair colors, consider the sphinx. For the really dark and bold-colored ladies, I suggest keeping that strip. Nothing looks sexier than a nice thick, black patch of hair with the perfect shape.

The other thing I like to consider before I make the decision, on which wax would look best on someone, is their body shape and anatomical shape. This may seem odd, but if you're a curvier woman, I have found, in my experience, that the more you leave behind, the better! I still suggest getting the labia, butt crack, and perianal areas waxed, but leave the wider strip or the extreme bikini shape behind. I have also noticed, in my experience, that my extremely petite women can feel a little uncomfortable with the sphinx because it can make them feel like they look even younger down there … you know what I mean!

Anatomically, there are all kinds of shapes and sizes. I will discuss this more through the chapters ahead, but I have noticed that if your labia/lip area is very pronounced, then getting the sphinx seems to be the most flattering. If your labia/lip area is very small and hidden, then leaving a little hair behind on this area looks a little better. Otherwise, what you do with the top part of the shape, whether it's the strip, the pie shape, or totally clean, seems to make little difference. However, with all these suggestions, nothing is sexier than feeling confident, so no matter what your shape or size, do what makes you feel your best.

Lastly, in considering which wax is best for you, I believe you need to think about your purpose and goal for your wax. If you know that you're the kind who will never want to be a long-term waxing person but want to surprise your significant other for a special event, or you're going on vacation and just want that once-a-year wax, then go for the gusto and get the sphinx or the Brazilian. I must say, this sort of guest is very rare; once you have experienced the smooth, sexy, and clean feeling of a wax, you will probably always want it that way.

Initially, my husband was the reason I got my first Brazilian wax. He'd been wanting me to go completely bare, but I was terrified of the pain. I'd had bikini waxes before—for "special occasions"—and couldn't imagine the pain of a Brazilian. It was a special occasion, along with my husband's pleading, that resulted in the first Brazilian. It was our three-year wedding anniversary and, in lieu of the honeymoon we never took after our wedding, we were going to Mexico to celebrate. I figured I could endure the pain for this special trip and always had in the back of my mind that, if it was too awful, I wouldn't have to do it again. It wasn't like my eyebrows that everyone sees, right? I mean, I don't have to wax down there. I'd do upkeep, of course, but I wasn't signing a contract that I'd forever go Brazilian. So I did it.

And the rest is history.

It still hurts—don't get me wrong. I sweat and pray for it to be over quickly. But I never regret having it done. It feels great. The silky smooth bare skin is wonderfully sensitive. It makes me feel sexy, and my husband is so appreciative. It's a win-win situation. With a small amount of pain for what you get in return.

Paige, 33, editor

I do have a few guests whom I only see once or twice a year, who can't wait to come in for their big annual waxes! If you know you want to become a regular waxer, then consider some of the suggestions I mentioned above, according to your hair type, shape, and most importantly, according to what will make you feel like a goddess!

Chapter 5
Making the Appointment

Okay, so hopefully you have decided to get a Brazilian wax done! Before you make an appointment at just any salon or spa, call around and ask the front reception desk a few questions.

1. First, ask if they have a licensed esthetician who performs Brazilian and sphinx waxes. Ask how many years of experience the esthetician has. Although I was good out of the gates, I, myself, would only go to a professional who has at least a few years of experience under their belt.

2. How long will the appointment take? If it is over twenty minutes, call another place. My Brazilians take me less than fifteen minutes to perform. A very good and experienced waxer will only need this amount of time. I have heard many horror stories of this procedure taking up to an hour! Some might tell you thirty minutes if it is your first time. I don't believe this is necessary for someone with good experience, but if you have heard good things about this waxer, then consider making the appointment.

3. Ask what type of wax they use. We will need to discuss this further, as many people have strong opinions about soft/warm and hard wax. Although hard wax is still warm to the touch, it is called hard wax since it hardens once it is laid on the skin. In my professional opinion and experience, nothing is better than soft wax. Hard wax claims to be more gentle; however, using this method of waxing is time-consuming, and the hair seems

to grow back faster, with many hairs breaking off during the procedure. In a hard wax treatment, they place a thick strip of wax on the area, let it cool, then pick at one end of the wax to pull up a little edge, then pull. Hard wax is done with many little strips and can get very painful. It is also in my experience that hard wax just doesn't pull up the hair as effectively as soft wax. I have had many regular guests who, after moving away or not being able to get into me, go to another spa and receive a hard-wax Brazilian; they return to me, sometimes driving over one hundred miles, because they are covered in, ingrown and broken-off hairs. It's just not worth possibly avoiding a tiny amount of pain. My opinion is if a waxer has been doing this for many years, they have seen how much more effective soft wax is.... Find an esthetician who uses soft wax, in my opinion.

4. Does the esthetician wear gloves? Believe it or not, there are many estheticians out there who do not wear gloves during the appointment. Gloves should obviously be worn for your safety and the esthetician's safety. And, on a personal note, I love wearing gloves because it makes me feel like I can touch any part of the guest that I might need to during the appointment! I am very thorough, and I like to make sure you go home with every inch clean and smooth. This might require me to hold one of your lips gently to the side, so I can get those hidden inner lip hairs! Gloves are just all-around necessary for hygiene and a professional experience.

5. Does the esthetician double-dip? Every single time the esthetician dips into the wax pot for wax, a new stick should be used. This is extremely important for your health and safety. If you ever see the esthetician double-dipping during your appointment, stop the procedure and leave. I have seen and heard of many estheticians who do not take this precaution, and it can be harmful to your health.

6. How much does the does a Brazilian cost? I will give you an estimate of how much you should expect to pay for each kind of wax. A standard bikini wax—twenty to twenty-five dollars.

Brazilian or sphinx—forty-five to sixty-five dollars. I charge forty-five dollars, but I know of many salons and spas that will charge up to sixty-five for the inclusion of the butt crack and perianal area. It is up to each esthetician and up to the salon's discretion. I have not heard of the charge going in excess of sixty-five dollars. The extreme bikini—thirty-five to forty dollars. As for the tip, anything from 10 percent to 20 percent is the normal rate. Sometimes I get more, and sometimes I get less. I realize that everyone's budget is different, so tip what you can afford and according to your experience.

7. You might want to ask the receptionist for the esthetician's name. This way, when you get to your appointment, you can tell them your name or the esthetician's. I also mention this because there are estheticians out there who are men, who do provide waxing services of this sort. I will say that I have known only one man who provided this service, and he was amazing. I have shared guests with him, who have gone to him for years and then start coming to me, and I have asked them what their experience was like with a male. I have heard both responses—that it did not make a difference, and he was fantastic at making them comfortable, or else many of my guests just did not feel comfortable with a man doing the service. That will have to be up to you, what you are okay with, but it's a good idea to ask the name, so you have the opportunity before your appointment to request a woman if you desire.

8. The reception desk might ask you if you are using anything from the dermatologist that might make you sensitive to wax, such as any Retin-A products or glycolic acids (although that would be highly unusual, and I have never heard of anyone using such products in the vaginal area), or if you are taking acne medications such as Accutane or Tetracycline. If they do not ask you this, you will be asked by your esthetician at your appointment, and if you are using any of these medications or topical treatments, then you can not be waxed. Please take this seriously; the top layer of your skin will come off. This could

leave you with an open sore and eventually a scab that could permanently scar.

These are a lot of question to ask the receptionist when you call around to figure out which salon or spa fits your needs, but once you find your place and your esthetician, you will develop a trusting, healthy, and professional relationship. It is possible the receptionist will not have an answer to all these questions, and you will decide to go anyways … and then you might notice they are not following any of these suggestions. Do not be afraid to stop the appointment and try another place. Make sure you feel absolutely safe and comfortable.

Chapter 6
How to Prepare for the Appointment

What can you do to prepare for the appointment once you have bravely booked your virgin wax? Clean yourself up for the esthetician. Take a nice, gentle shower, and soap up the area and rinse well. I do not recommend a bath. I have had several guests who soaked before coming, and the skin is so pliable and warm that it is too sensitive to work on. If you don't have time to shower before the appointment, use a baby wipe, feminine cloth, or gently wipe the area with a washcloth. I keep saying gentle for a reason! I can tell that some guests have rubbed the area so aggressively that they are red and sensitive. Be kind to yourself! Clean and wipe out your inner lip and labia area. It is amazing to me what I see sometimes! I understand that, as women, we all have times of the month when we are a little juicier, with excess discharge. But bringing a wipe or cloth and using it right before your appointment will make a better experience for both of us. Look at yourself, and get comfortable with how beautiful your vagina is … and take good care of it. Open the lips and labia, and use your fingers to gently wipe out this inner area. Spread those butt cheeks apart, and wipe or rinse yourself. Prepare your vagina for its goddess work!

Please do not go to a tanning bed the day before or the day of your appointment. It is a good idea to avoid the tanning bed a few days after also. If you're getting ready for a big event like a wedding and must tan, then do it the day before in the morning, and be extra gentle to your sweet spot! And then wait a day after the waxing before going back to the tanning bed. Your skin will be extremely sensitive during this time, and a little rawness or bruising could happen.

There is so much confusion by my guests about how long the hair should be. I tell everyone to let it get as long and wild as they can grow it! There is way more potential for not being able to perform the wax if the hair is too short, because the wax will not grab too-short hair. And if we decide to go through with doing the wax, there is more possibility for bruising and a painful experience with shorter hair. I always appreciate when my guests want to tidy up the area and groom it a little for me … but just leave it alone. I would rather trim it for you and know that it is the proper length than send you home without a wax, or bruise you. If you are growing it out, and you're an avid shaver, please give it several weeks, I know this is difficult for those of you who are not used to having hair, but it will be well worth the couple of weeks of growing it out. A quarter of an inch of outgrowth is the minimum—I like to say, about the length of an eyebrow or arm hair. My favorite is someone who lets it go for an entire month and comes in with a giant bush! It's more work for me, but I know that you will go home with a perfect Brazilian!

For your first time receiving your virgin Brazilian wax, you might want to consider booking your appointment a week after your menstrual cycle. The week prior to menstruation and during it can make the experience more painful. Your sensitivity is physically and emotionally heightened, so plan it around your normal cycle. I will discuss this topic more thoroughly later in the coming chapters, but if you are waxing for a special event, and the only time you are able to wax is during your cycle, then you can still safely receive a wax job.

Another helpful suggestion is to gently exfoliate the area for several days before your wax. You don't need to exfoliate the lips, labia, or butt crack. Focus on the area in your leg crease and the actual muff! Exfoliating will help lift the dead skin and open the follicles so the hair is easier to remove and will also help avoid ingrown hairs (we will confront this topic more in depth later!). Again, be gentle and kind to yourself. Use a loofah with a gentle soap, or a washcloth will work just as well. It doesn't take much for this area to exfoliate properly.

I am amazed at how much my final suggestion helps with preventing bruising and irritation: *Do not* wear underwear! I tell my ladies, if they can help it, to try not to wear anything tight or constricting for the whole day before their appointment. Even if you can sneak your panties off the hour before you come in, it seems to help. Try to plan your outfit for the day of your wax to be something loose and comfortable. If you have the luxury of coming from home the day of your appointment, then wear a skirt or sweat pants. I have noticed through the years that the elastic band that rests against the outside bikini line puts pressure on this sensitive spot. This spot, where the thigh meets the vagina, is where most people bruise. The nerve that runs down the inside of your thigh is supplied by a huge amount of blood right at the surface, and most people's skin is very thin in that area. Try to keep any constriction or pressure away from there if possible … it will help prevent bruising! And, yes, you will not be wearing your underwear during the procedure. Some salons offer a disposable thong to wear if you're feeling shy, but this will only get in the way of the areas I want to wax. But if you're just getting a regular bikini wax, wear something that is small and loose enough that we can still negotiate around and do not wear your favorite pair. Wax can go flying, and sometimes a little might get stuck to the side of your underwear—another reason that you should throw your shyness to the wind and just plan on coming in and taking it all off! It will make it easier on us both in the end.

As for taking something to prevent pain before you come in … some people are so nervous their first time that they feel they must take a pain-reliever. I have very few regulars who take something before their appointment. But if you are very worried about the pain, you can take a couple ibuprofen or aspirin an hour before your appointment. I have a couple guests who swear by taking an ibuprofen with an antacid to help with the pain and redness. I have not experienced this to make a huge difference in the service, but I'm giving you all the information I have ever heard or experienced. Although I do not recommend this next suggestion, I have several guests who swear by taking a shot of tequila or drinking a glass of wine before the appointment. This definitely will relax you, but alcohol of any kind is not helpful for the pain or redness, and it will make you more red and sensitive, if anything. I have one guest whom I have been waxing for many years, and through trial and error, we have discovered if she drinks a cup of coffee and eats a banana, she feels less sensitive and has an easier recovery time. Again, I can't swear by or guarantee that any of these before-treatments will make the pain less or the experience better, but they are tools and ideas that can and are being used!

Chapter 7
What to Expect at Your First Appointment

Now that you have made the appointment and have been gently exfoliating for the last couple of days, your big day is here for your first virgin wax! Don't be nervous; you will only create more problems with the anticipation of what it might be like. Most guests tell me at the end, that the pain and the experience were not nearly as terrible as they had set themselves up for.

I am one of those people who will try anything once, so I got a Brazilian wax. Now I would not go back. Having nothing in the way makes me feel sexy in my clothes, not to mention the added pleasure it gives in compromising positions. I don't need to check my bikini line when I get in a bathing suit. There is nothing like a bare vagina to entice an appetite, not to mention how it feels for you! Did it hurt? Um, hello … yes … but in the long run, not more than several Band-Aids being peeled off in succession and a bit of a therapeutic hot feeling for a few hours afterwards. Now it is just part of the process, not something to be feared.

Tanya, 36, computer technician

I was in Brazil, and my Brazilian buddy had told the esthetician what wax job to do. So there I was, on the table, legs open, a Brazilian bikini wax virgin, thinking she'd just clean up the sides. Next thing I feel, she's applying hot wax to my outer labia and ready to roll. I arch my back off the table as the pain from ripping blows through my body. Nobody told me what to expect! But after it was over, I realized how awesome it truly was to not have a lick of hair covering my nani. I hate hair. I'm East Indian, and we're a hairy breed! I was smooth for weeks! There was no itchiness, like after shaving, and no thick, pokey hairs growing in the next day. And, the cherry on top was that, in the weeks to follow, I wore my little Brazilian bikini with such confidence, knowing there was no way a stray hair was peeking out the sides of my minimal-coverage swimsuit. Some people get it done for their boyfriend, and that's only 20 percent of my reason. He loves it and cannot wait for a newly waxed nani. He even likes to imagine a girl waxing me down there, so I let him imagine, even though it's far from pornography. I simply love it because the benefits of a smooth, clean, noncluttered nani far outweigh the three minutes of ripping. I wish for everyone to join the world of Brazilian waxing. It's really not that bad, and well worth the moment of pain. I've been doing it diligently every one to two months for seven years, and I'd rather hold out for a waxer than go back to shaving. *Thank you, Brazil!*

Reena, 28, vet student

Start to get yourself excited for the results! How smooth, sexy, and clean it is going to feel down there when the waxing is over and for weeks to come. Start to see yourself as the amazing goddess you are— you are going to become one of those sheik women with a secret in her panties that drives her partner wild!,

Once you have checked in at the front desk for your appointment, ask to use the restroom. This is your opportunity to do any last-minute cleanup, in case you're coming to your appointment straight from work, shopping, or such. Some places, especially waxing-only places, will provide wipes for the vaginal area in the restroom. If not, you may have remembered to bring your own ... and just gently wipe the area with a paper towel. Again, I emphasize the importance of being kind to yourself always, but definitely right before your appointment—you don't want to aggravate the skin. Pull the lips apart, and softly wipe out the labia, perianal area, and inner vagina. Prepare your canvas for your artist!

Your esthetician will come out and call your name and introduce herself. You will follow her back to her private room in the spa. If you have not used the restroom and have blanked that suggestion out, the esthetician will usually ask you on the way back if you need to use the restroom. Once you enter the esthetician's room, you will see a massage table or cot of some sort with a clean sheet lying over the top. A disposable thong underwear or a towel for you to put over your lap may be provided. The esthetician will then ask you a few questions. She will want to know when your last Brazilian was or if this is your first time. She will ask if you are taking any medications or topical treatments that might make your skin sensitive to waxing. This is also your opportunity to ask any questions you might have, and don't forget you are paying for this service, so make sure you feel completely comfortable.

Look around the room, and make sure it looks clean and professional. You should begin to feel a connection with your esthetician immediately. I feel half of what you're paying for is the expertise and experience of a professional who knows the awkward position you are in and will put you at ease immediately! Once you have answered the esthetician's questions and have had any of your questions answered, the esthetician will ask you to take your pants and underwear off and get up on top of the sheet on the table. At this point, you can put on the disposable thong or use a towel over your waist if you're feeling shy. Many of my fellow estheticians will leave the room after these instructions, so you can undress and prepare by yourself. I, however, don't leave the room. I'm going to see it all anyways, and I feel that I'm establishing more comfort by staying in the room with you. In my opinion, this is a team effort from start to finish, and I can keep the conversation going during the entire experience if I stay. I have also noticed that even my long-time guests forget what to take off and what to do when they come in, so I find it is easier to just stay in the room. But expect either possibility at your appointment.

I am going to explain what happens next, the way I perform my Brazilian waxes, but I will also explain the other ways some estheticians do their Brazilians. Of course, I believe my way is the most effective, as

I have tried every position possible, but I want you to be prepared for anything and everything! Once you're up on the table and undressed, I ask you to put the soles of your feet together and spread your knees apart like a frog lady, so you are wide open, lying on the table with everything exposed. Depending on your flexibility, I will have you scoot your butt down toward your feet to get a wider stretch. If your flexibility is limited, I will have you keep your feet farther from your butt so your knees lay a little flatter toward the table. If your flexibility is extremely limited, and it hurts your hips to lay this way at all, I find that rolling up a separate sheet or tucking a small pillow under each hip really helps with any discomfort in the hip region. You will be in this starting position for most of the wax. I will only have you change positions once at the very end for the last two strips of hair in the perianal area. Now, for the alternate positions some estheticians may use. They may have you bring only one leg up at a time, so the sole of one of your feet is resting against the inside of the opposite leg's knee. Although this position may seem less invasive and less embarrassing at first, it makes it more difficult for the esthetician to really get in to the labia and inner lip area. You will not get as clean a wax job. Open up those legs, and spread it all open! It may seem weird at first, but you are paying a lot of money to get a good, clean wax, so open up and let us in, so we can do our job!

Now that we have you half-naked and hopefully lying in the frog-lady position with your beautiful self totally exposed, the wax job can really begin. The esthetician will put on a fresh pair of sterile gloves and look over the area to be waxed. Hopefully, you have been growing in the hair for a couple weeks, and my ultimate favorite is when you have never groomed, and you have a full seventies bush—these folks really get the shock of their lives! If your hair is a little too long, the hair will be trimmed slightly. Remember—the longer the hair, the better.

Now, this final preparation is different for each esthetician, so I will tell you my favorite technique but will also share what else to expect. (Here we go. I'm letting out my tightly held trade secrets to all those other estheticians!) Most estheticians will lay a little baby powder or skin prep solution down on the skin of the area to be waxed. My favorite is to put a little jojoba oil on the labia and inner lip area. Jojoba oil most easily matches the natural oil of skin and allows the hair to still come out from the root, but keeps the wax from pulling up any thin skin in this most precious and sensitive of areas. Other than on the lip area, I do not apply oil or anything on the rest of the bikini area. I have noticed that, although powder may help a *little* with the pain, it can keep some of the roots from fully coming up, thus not allowing a perfect and clean wax. Some estheticians will use nothing at all. Again, once you find the esthetician who loves her job and takes it very seriously, you will want and expect her to really get in there.... I put a little oil on my gloved fingers, open up the labia, and really get in there, to make sure I have you fully covered with oil. If I'm shy and nervous, then we really won't get anywhere! Either way, expect some sort of preparation before the wax is laid on the skin.

Now the real fun begins! I start with the outside bikini area first. I have found that most, if not all, estheticians will start with the outside of the bikini area and work their way in, doing the labia and perianal area last. Using a fresh stick every time, I will dip the stick in the pot and scoop up a layer of wax. I will smooth warm wax onto the area in the direction of your natural hair growth. I have had guests tell me they were concerned that the wax would feel too hot. The wax will feel warm and maybe a little warmer once we reach the inner lip area but should never feel hot. I am a speed waxer, so I may dip a new stick in the pot and lay the warm wax on several areas. Some estheticians may do one strip at a time, so be prepared for either method of laying the wax down. A cloth strip is laid over the wax, and the esthetician will either press on the strip of cloth or rub it gently a few times before pulling. The esthetician should hold the skin taut on the opposite side of where she is getting ready to pull the strip of cloth. Another perfect example of why gloves are so necessary is that sometimes the part of skin I'm holding may be close to the lip and labia area, and if I want to get a good firm grip, I want to feel comfortable touching whatever I might need to in order to keep pain to a minimum. The esthetician will pull the strip at an angle away from the body. The pull should be a nice, smooth, but very fast pull. If the pull is done too slowly, it will stick to the body and be extremely painful. If the pull is done straight up, away from the body rather than at an angle, you risk bruising. Right after the strip of cloth is pulled; the esthetician will take her free hand and apply pressure to the spot that was just waxed. The purpose for applying pressure is that the nerve receptors for pain and pressure are the same. So, if you have pain and pressure happening at the same time in the same spot, they compete with one another. If the brain circuit is busy with pressure, it can't transmit pain! This technique of laying the wax and using a cloth strip to pull the hair out, followed by pressure, will be done while working our way in toward the center goddess spot.

Most estheticians, including myself, will also do the inner thigh area where those pesky hairs grow down toward your knees! Once the outside bikini area is done, it's time for everyone's most anticipated labia and lip area. I hold the labia open and lay the wax over the spot I have oiled in the direction of the hair growth … sometimes this requires me to get my face really up close and personal, to investigate just which direction those sneaky hairs are growing! I like to hold the lip area myself, but I know many estheticians who will ask you to hold your own lip to the side while they apply the wax. After laying the wax, I apply the cloth strip and have the guest take a deep breath in and exhale. As you exhale, I pull the strip away from your body, removing the lip hairs. I have so many jokes about trying to get the guest to exhale properly; it makes me laugh still when I say them. Most people are so nervous that their attempts to exhale are short and cut off. My favorite serious but funny joke is to tell them to exhale so hard they blow my hair off my face! My guests who practice yoga or have just had a baby tend to be the best at the inhale-and-exhale. Although this breathing does help a little with the pain, it really just helps release the nervousness, and it gives you something else to focus on … because I promise you that, although this is your scariest place to have waxed, it truly is the least painful. The most painful is the spot right above your clitoris; that is why leaving a landing strip of hair is recommended. I like to call this tough spot "the Hitler," because it looks like a little Hitler mustache when it's left behind, and this area is the most painful to get waxed!

Once the lip area is done, it's time to move into the second position. This is another one of those secrets that I know not many estheticians know about, so I will tell you how I do the perianal area, and I will tell you what to possibly expect. I have you bring your knees to your chest, fold your arms under your knees, and pull as tight as you can. Most estheticians have the guest turn over and get on all fours. There is one other position that I may use if you are pregnant—I have you turn on your side. I have noticed during my time that people are very thankful for my positions, because they make the whole experience seem less embarrassing and less invasive. I also have noticed that in the knees-to-chest position, the skin is nice and taut in the butt cheek and perianal areas. So, the butt cheeks naturally open up, and I can get in there! Please don't be embarrassed about this final part of the wax. It is most people's favorite area of hair to have removed. There is minimal pain, and it would look strange to have a clean vagina and a hairy butt! I have some guests who have come to me for years who still nervously laugh when we do this section. I will admit that even I feel funny getting it done, but it is so worth it! Not every esthetician will do the butt crack area, but when you find a professional who loves her work and knows how great it is to have that hair gone, you will be pleased. The same procedure is used in this area, of laying the wax and pulling with a cloth strip, followed by pressure. Most experienced estheticians, including myself, will follow the wax job with a small amount of tweezing of any hairs left behind.

After the entire area is waxed and tweezed, the esthetician will put something on the area to help cool it down and get it on the road to healing. I like to use the jojoba oil with a cloth to make sure no wax is left behind on the skin. There is nothing more annoying than going home feeling sticky in your crotch! There are many different types of post-waxing solutions out there, but I have found jojoba oil to be the best, as it helps restore the oil on the skin that was removed, helps with wax residue, and gets the skin on its way to healing faster.

Sometimes if a guest is extremely susceptible to ingrown hairs, I will apply a thin layer of salicylic acid after applying the oil. Either way, expect the esthetician to apply some sort of topical treatment after the wax job is complete. I like to apply the after-treatment myself, as I can usually see what you can't. Some estheticians might hand you a cloth with the topical treatment for you to apply to yourself, so be prepared for either scenario. I like to hand my guests a mirror so they can see what they look like all cleaned up; this is one of those moments when I feel that true goddess work comes into play.

The first time I went in to get a Brazilian wax, I was mortified. By the time the job was done, I was in love with Molly and my newly discovered private parts! She really got me thinking and realizing that maybe I am normal-looking down there. That it's not this fleshy thing, only to be used in the dark…She made me look at it in the mirror after! Immediately, I noticed that my newly waxed area was sooo soft that even a breeze felt exciting! I must admit that I only got the wax because I wanted to feel cleaner and tidier, but I was the most surprised. I could feel things like I had never felt before. I was juicier and able to orgasm so much easier … I couldn't believe it! I enjoy looking at myself now and no longer see my vagina as ugly. I always want it clean, but when it's time for my appointment, I know I will be staring at myself and having the best sex for the upcoming few weeks. Incredible.

Jody, 33, teacher

I have so many guests who don't care to look, and I usually make them! I have others who take the mirror and carefully examine every inch and even touch the freshly waxed area to make sure it feels smooth and I didn't miss a spot. The first time you look at yourself totally hairless, you can have many reactions. Some people just stare at themselves like it is the first time they have ever really seen themselves, others smile and get excited to be clean, and then there are the ones I discussed before, who want nothing to do with it … I'm still working on you ladies to love, know, appreciate, and enjoy your beautiful, fantastic vaginas!

You can get up and get dressed at this point. Again, I usually do not leave the room, but some estheticians will leave the room for you to get dressed privately. Your esthetician will walk you up to the front desk and will usually recommend you prebook your next appointment. She will generally discuss aftercare and might recommend some products for you to purchase.

Chapter 8
Now What? Aftercare

You have successfully received and completed your first Brazilian! You might feel a little sore for one or two days. Some guests are only uncomfortable for a few hours, and even the worst soreness never lasts longer than a day or two. During my first few months of getting waxed, I felt sore for two days, but today I'm ready to go and feel comfortable within twenty minutes.

If you have not touched your new found cave in the room right after your appointment, the first thing you need to do is touch it! The first time I got mine, I could not keep my hands off of myself. Not in any sexual way, of course, but it felt sooo soft. Please feel yourself after the appointment; it is the softest, most velvety skin you have ever touched. You must look at it closely too ... there are no black nubs of hair under the skin, just smooth, clear, and amazing skin. Right after your wax job, you will find yourself feeling a little different already. An extra strut in your walk, an air of confidence and an oozing sexiness, knowing what lies ahead. You have just opened yourself up to a whole new lifestyle of really knowing yourself ... you have gotten a taste of goddess work at its best!

Firstly, I recommend prebooking your next appointment while you're leaving. Most estheticians will advise this upon your leaving after your appointment. The standard for your next appointment that I recommend is to schedule it four or five weeks later. There are usually, in most humans, three growth cycles of hair. It takes four weeks for at least one of the growth cycles to take place. Everyone is different, but for the first two or three weeks, you are in love with me for changing your life. Around week three, the first growth cycle will begin to show, you will notice a few stray soft hairs starting to grow. You may not even notice the hairs. Yes, ladies, the hair that grows back after a wax is so soft that you may not even notice the hairs. At about three to four weeks, you're starting to think about me and about getting another goddess treatment. By week five, the second growth cycle begins to come through and you can't wait to get into your next appointment and are feeling extremely happy that you prebooked, so you know for sure you will be seeing me and will not have to wait. Again, everyone is different. If your hair is extremely coarse and difficult, I might recommend your next appointment to be at four weeks. Either way, waxing is a team effort and we will discover together what amount of time between waxing works best for you. Also, as time goes on with dedicated waxing, the time between needing waxed will lengthen. I have guests who once needed to come in every four weeks that now can stay smooth up to eight weeks at a time between waxings. And those famous movie stars I discussed earlier were regulars who received their treatments every two weeks. But let me explain further that if our ultimate goal is to destroy the hair follicle, then we need a minimum of one growth cycle and ultimately two growth cycles. You will be smooth longer if you can wait more time for those hairs to come back in. If you can afford it and never want a trace of hair, then consider going more often, but it is not my personal recommendation. Trust the advice of your waxing professional for when to book your next appointment; if she is truly experienced, she will consider your hair type, personality, pain tolerance, and goals.

For most guests, ingrown hairs are not an issue. For these lucky individuals, I recommend after your waxing job to just go home, and if you're not already wearing something loose and comfortable, go home as soon as possible and put something happy on! For the first night, you want to air it out. Leave the jojoba oil or post-waxing solution that your esthetician applied, on your new wax overnight. For the next couple of days when you bathe, just clean the area gently with a mild soap. Use *no* lotions or potions after you shower! Just wash kindly and pat dry. If you want to exfoliate the area after a few weeks to get ready for your next appointment, that would be great, but do it nicely and softly.

Now for the heavy topic of the ever-annoying ingrown hair! An ingrown hair is a hair that curls back around and penetrates the skin with its tip. Once this hair penetrates the skin, it causes an eruption or inflammation, followed by pus, redness, and itchiness. Even writing about it makes my skin crawl; I have been battling this with my guests for years. Although the possibility of an ingrown hair is less common with waxing than shaving, it still haunts many of my guests. Most ingrown hairs will heal by themselves without any treatment; however, there are many solutions to this enemy that I have discovered through the years. I have to admit that several of my guests have been my guinea pigs during the years, and I have found what works and what does not. For those few ingrown hairs that might follow a wax—everyone might get one or two—just let them heal on their own. Please do not try to do mini-surgery at home; picking and squeezing the hair will not help. Most ingrown hair sufferers are those with very curly and coarse hair. First of all, do not exfoliate the skin with anything aggressive such as a scrub or loofah, because it will only cause more irritation. However, there are several different effective approaches one can take. First, you might need to try letting the hair grow a little longer before your next waxing appointment. This is one of those moments when coming too often can cause an issue, and letting the hair get longer will help. I recommend using a topical acne treatment such as salicylic acid to gently exfoliate the skin and kill bacteria. Just go get some medicated facial acne pads from the grocery store—the kind that one would use as a daily wipe on facial acne. There are several different brands out there you can purchase, but just make sure they contain salicylic acid. I tell my guests to begin wiping the area with one of these pads every day for the first three to four days after their wax job, and then just swipe the area a couple times a week until their next appointment. My few guests who suffer from many ingrown hairs can consider using an after-shave treatment designed for ingrown hairs, which can be purchased from a beauty outlet store. These topical creams are made for men to use on their faces after shaving. There are very few people who will need to hunt out this sort of treatment, because most people find the salicylic pads to be very effective. I favor the pads because they are convenient and because they have no smell. I have found that many of my guests complain about the after-shave creams because they leave a residue and smell bad. Over time, the combination of waxing and using the pads will decrease your ingrown hairs.

There are so many topical after-wax treatments being sold right now, and your esthetician may recommend one of these options. I have found that most of these are expensive and are usually too strong for most guests. Most of them burn when you put them on, and if they are too strong, they will only worsen the issue by causing more irritation. Trust the advice of your esthetician, but consider the salicylic acid pads, as they have proven to be the best defense against ingrown hairs, in my experience.

There are a few people, and it seems to be mostly my redheads, who have that lily-white, sensitive skin that just gets plain-old irritated. Although I have seen this in all types of hair and skin, it took me a while to realize that they were not suffering from ingrown hairs but from irritation. One of my usual guests had the worst case of what we thought were ingrown hairs. She came to me regularly for years and used all the treatments out there with perfect discipline. During one of her appointments, we both could not believe how clear and calm her skin looked. She said she had run out of all the treatments and was not able to use anything … we were both confused. Then I had another guest with a similar story who ran out of all her products but found some hydrocortisone cream in her closet and decided on her own to give it a whirl. We both could not believe how calm and clear her skin looked. So the experiments began. I started recommending aloe vera and hydrocortisone to my guests who had constant irritation and seemed to fit the criteria. It was such a miracle for me and these women to find an easy solution! I will never stop learning from my guests; they have been my best teachers. So, if you are covered in tiny little red bumps, besides the normal inflamed ones that occur for the first few hours after your wax, consider trying aloe vera or hydrocortisone for the first few days after your appointment.

If you feel that you have something more intense going on, and none of these suggestions help, please call your esthetician or make an appointment so you may work together to resolve the issue.

Now, for the most important aftercare advice I can give. *Do not shave!* I could write novels about how many of my guests have learned their lesson on this one. I understand that during the first few months you start to wax, the hair is still growing in strong, but if you can just get through the first three consecutive wax jobs without shaving, then you will be hooked for life. After your first appointment, you will notice that the hair is softer and a little less thick, but after the third one, you have usually successfully started to destroy the follicles. Every time you shave, you slice the hair off at the base, and it leaves a thick, flat nub under the surface of your skin, so when that hair starts to grow back, the tip is thick and strong. This is why the ingrown hairs from shaving are the very worst and hardest to treat. It is also why the hair is so coarse, itchy, and angry! However, when you wax the hair and remove the root, the hair naturally grows back in at a thin angle, leaving you with soft, thin regrowth, without the itchy, coarse aftermath from shaving. For my guests who are outdoors in a swimsuit most of the year, I tell them to go buy a cute boy-short swimsuit for that one week before their next appointment when the hairs are starting to show.

Another reason I am against shaving is a personal opinion. The whole reason I discovered waxing is because I used to be a raging hippie! Back in the day, I was fully grown in—my legs, underarms, and bush hair were my symbol and testament that grooming was not part of my true beauty, and no man was going to put me through such an unnecessary task! I was still under the belief that hair removal was for them, not me … but more importantly, I was green before it was cool to be green. Before I decided to let it all grow, I went through razors and blades every week like most of us do, and I couldn't stand all the garbage that came with shaving. It seemed cruel to the environment and to my precious time. But during that one fateful summer that brought me here, I decided I wanted my legs back and began looking for an alternative to shaving. I went to my first wax appointment for a full leg wax. She just kept on going up my leg until she asked if I wanted my bikini done as well … and it changed my life—obviously! Suddenly, there was a environmentally healthy alternative to hair removal, and I became obsessed with how smooth and good it felt to be hairless. And the bikini wax made me feel like I was reborn! So to that hippie guy I dated in college who thought I needed grooming, I apologize, and you should have waited a little longer! So, it's well worth the wait between appointments to have a little hair, in order to work toward your goal of being a Brazilian waxing goddess!

Chapter 9
Embarrassing Questions Answered!

This chapter is the reason I decided to write this little manual. It's amazing to me how many questions I repeatedly get asked, whether it's by a guest in the room getting an actual Brazilian wax, or at a barbecue by a stranger once he or she finds out what I do, or by my mother's card club, by friends whom I have known since childhood, or even by men who really want to know what is going on in there! Just recently, a guest of mine who is a surgeon admitted to me that during surgery, there were four women helping with the procedure and, of the five ladies, two were also my guests. The other nonwaxers were asking them a million questions during surgery! It takes people a minute to feel comfortable asking, but once they have broken the seal of questioning, it is incredible what everyone wants to know. They want to know the truth. There are so many guests who have inspired me to get this kind of information out there.

There was one woman in her fifties who had just returned from a vacation with her girlfriends. She had always wanted to get a Brazilian and had started asking questions about what her girlfriend's thought about getting waxed. She told me she felt ridiculous trying to get a conversation going about this subject, because they made her feel like it was taboo or inappropriate to discuss. Once she finally decided to come in, I could tell she was just dying to ask me a hundred questions. She has been a regular for several years now, and she still has questions for me every time she comes in. My mother, who is almost seventy and an avid quilter and card player, told her friends after years of keeping it under wraps because she wasn't even entirely sure what I did! And suddenly the same questions started flowing in from these cute little grandmas who had been in mystery about this subject for their whole lives but had no one to ask.

I love what I do … I keep saying this for a reason. I have watched so much body healing and vagina healing take place in my room, and it is beautiful. I have worked very hard to create a space where women can talk, ask, admire, and find the goddess within themselves. And opening up the forum for talking about this issue has created many interesting conversations with groups of people from every walk of life. I love what I do … I have had groups of women at the bar, wide-eyed and thankful, filled with questions. I love what I do … I have had women of every age group relax in front of the mirror and gaze at their beauty with love for the first time. I love what I do … I have given women who thought they looked funny or different down there, the insight that everyone looks unique, and no one looks funny. I love what I do … I have heard countless stories of couples that have renewed their sex lives through this simple act of goddess work. I love what I do …

I met my younger friend for a drink one night, which is rare for me, and after a few margaritas, she shared that she had just gotten a Brazilian wax to spice up her sex life. I grilled her with questions, and I guess I had never known that you could wax your pussy and have it grow back soft. To tell you the truth, she was turning me on. I had tried shaving, and that was so horrible when it grew back. After that night, I called right away to get an appointment. I thought I could wait a month for my twenty-fifth anniversary, but I couldn't wait. I set up a surprise date for that night, not telling my husband what it was Now I realize the hot date should have been a day later, but still he was so excited. Well, was I ever pleased. I had never felt that my pussy was pretty, just a hairy thing down there, but with a Brazilian, I felt like my pussy was pretty, and I pranced around showing it off wearing little pieces of lingerie tempting my husband, and my sex life was great for weeks even after it started to grow out. My husband ate me out all the time, which hardly ever used to happen that, is why I continue to get Brazilians. What better thing to spend money on than good sex

- celebrate yourself, celebrate sex, be beautiful inside, outside, and down there … it feels so soft.

Leslie, 48, carpenter

So, although I thought it necessary to explain every process that goes into getting a Brazilian wax, the following sections are the most asked questions that everyone is really dying to know!.

Farting

Let's start with the really embarrassing thing first. Everyone eventually admits to me that they're afraid they're going to fart! Let's use the word fart, since I will not be able to keep using elegant words for it during the entire paragraph, and you already know my style is one of gritty realness. It has only happened twice during my entire profession. But, yes, it has happened! The first time I was farted on, and, yes, it was square in the face, was by a woman who had just had surgery down there. The skin of the perianal area was very loose and open, plus, because of the surgery, she was extremely gassy. She was mortified, and she started crying and was completely humiliated and apologetic. Hey, you know what? I'm a human being who farts accidentally too! I reassured her that it was a completely normal human situation that could happen to anyone. When I get my Brazilian, the thought crosses my mind, too, that one might slip out.

The second time was a very regular guest of mine, and it was actually kind of funny. Once I put her into position two with the knees to the chest, a little one squeaked out. She suddenly started talking really loudly about I don't even know what! I wanted to laugh—trust me, I thought it was funny but wanted to respect her dignity and realized she wanted to pretend it didn't happen. So I kept waxing her, and she kept talking louder, and the farting continued in little short bursts. We all react in different ways to embarrassing situations. I probably would laugh but feel terrible for my esthetician. However, there is no need to feel bad; those of us who have been doing this for a long time are very comfortable with the body and its functions. We understand that we're all human, and these things happen. There is also a global understanding that farts can happen, and sometimes we pretend they didn't happen, but other times, we nervously laugh it off. She still comes to me for her regular Brazilian, and neither of us has ever mentioned it. It actually makes me feel good about myself that she feels comfortable with me enough to know that I would never think differently of her. That is two occurrences of farts in over ten years of waxing, so please don't let this silly and common fear hold you back from getting waxed. It probably will never happen to you. And if you are not feeling well and are really nervous about the possibility of one blasting out of you, then reschedule your appointment. And if by some crazy voodoo, you are one of the rare people whom it might happen to once, then react however you want. Laugh, apologize, or just keep talking like it didn't happen, and guide us in how you want the situation treated. Professionals in this trade are prepared for these situations, and we're totally aware that it can happen anytime!

Menstrual Cycle

Let's discuss the possibility of having your menstrual cycle during your scheduled appointment. I have to be honest that I'm not sure how many estheticians are comfortable with performing your wax during your period. It is in my opinion, however, that a true professional with a lot of experience has run into this possibility as often as I have and feels fine doing it. Try to schedule your first wax during a time when you will not have your cycle, just to be safe, and then once you have built a relationship with your esthetician, ask her how she feels about it.

Although, as we discussed earlier, your skin sensitivity and pain tolerance will be heightened during your menstrual cycle, I still have at least one guest a day who is on her period who is scheduled and doesn't want to miss her appointment. I am totally comfortable with doing a wax during this sacred time, but I prefer to do the wax while you're wearing a tampon. I will wax you if you're not able to wear a tampon, but it's not as easy. So how do I do it? I just place the tampon string on one side of the labia while I wax one side, then switch it over and tuck inside the lip on the other side while I finish the other inner lip area. No problem, no big deal. I have never gotten wax on a tampon string and ripped it out … I know that's what you're wondering right now! It has never happened and never will. I am completely aware of where the string is the entire time I'm doing the wax job. I'm not grossed out or feeling weird in anyway whatsoever ... I said it before, and I will say it many times throughout this chapter. Guess what? I'm a human being, too, who deals with her period every month and manages to touch her own tampon with ease, so yours is no big deal. It's all the same stuff going on down there, and we need to start feeling comfortable about it and discussing it openly. So, if you're needing a wax, and it's your time of the month, then ask your esthetician how she feels about waxing during this time. Someone with experience will have no problem performing the job.

Does Sex Feel Different after Getting a Brazilian Wax?

I have one big, wonderful answer to this question—yes!!! From my own experience and all of my beautiful guests' experiences, I can say that you will feel much more sensitive, soft, and hyperaware in your goddess zone. Another little interesting result is that you are much wetter and juicier after the wax.

> I walked into my first appointment with Molly, fully expecting to get a bikini wax. Well, within thirty seconds of meeting her, she had me talked into a Brazilian ... *eeek!* I was nervous, because I had no idea what I was getting myself into, but I just kept reminding myself what Molly told me that sold me on the idea ... sex would be better than I ever had it; who would turn that down, right? Well, the girl didn't lie! It's seriously never been better; I feel *everything* during sex now and get wet faster than ever in my life ... I love it and can't imagine going back to my old ways!
>
> Anna, 36, software sales executive

All that stiff pubic hair held your moisture and after removing this block, you are free-flowing. Many women, especially in menopause, lose some of this wetness and lubrication. They find, after the hair is gone, that there is much more glide and sensation. The feedback I get from clients about their partners' experience with them after the wax is that the partners love the extra juice and the softness. Another interesting piece of feedback I get is that oral sex is suddenly an entirely new experience. Whether it's the excitement of the partner experiencing a totally clean canvas to enjoy or the new sensations the woman is feeling, I'm not sure, as I've heard both! So that is the physical experience ... but let's consider the visual experience of the guest and her partner! I have had the distinct honor of hearing stories from clients about their husbands being speechless when they see their suddenly new sexy goddesses, and the two of them experience the greatest night of lovemaking of their lives! A Brazilian will make sex physically feel better, but the most important thing in improving your sex life is feeling sexy about yourself. A Brazilian wax physically and visually will definitely shake things up in the bedroom and give you a whole new appreciation for your body!

> I decided to get my first Brazilian for a Valentine's Day present for my husband. After being married for five years, I was running out of sexy, romantic ideas. I nervously scheduled my first appointment but was pleasantly surprised when it hurt slightly less than childbirth. On Valentine's night, it didn't matter, the pain or discomfort that I had gone through. The rose petal stains on the comforter tell the story. Now, I willingly and excitedly schedule each appointment knowing how good I will feel afterwards. Having a nice, clean "muffin," as we like to call it, makes me feel sexy and confident, in and out of the bedroom. It is something that my husband and I both enjoy and look forward to each month. I love to see the look on his face each time I get home. It is like a kid in a candy store, and I am happy to sell whatever he wants to buy.
>
> Paula, (age not included), wife/mother/speech therapist

Smell

Okay, let's keep delving even further into those embarrassing topics that you're dying to know—we'll go right into smell. This is one of those questions that I most often get from people outside of the waxing room. However, I have had several guests who, after feeling totally comfortable with me, ask if they have a scent to them or if they smell bad. They always say "bad" ... that's the question I get. Is the smell bad?

Of course, there is usually a little bit of a scent, but never, ever, never bad! Come on, people; we have to stop associating our natural beautiful vaginas with anything bad! Do I really need to keep lecturing everyone about how amazing we are? Well, I know I do, because this topic comes up every day. Some people just can't believe what I do, because they are so afraid of the idea of smelling another human's essence. Or a guest will shyly ask if she smells worse than my usual guests. Guess what? I'm going to repeat myself. If there is a smell, then you smell just like me, a human being. There is nothing foul or weird about it; it's natural and perfect. We know our bodies, usually, as women, and there are certain times of the month when we are a little gooier with extra discharge, and I know what I'm seeing when I see that. However, using my suggestion of bringing some sanitary wipes to use right before your appointment will avoid the possibility of this happening. I can tell that some guests have sprayed perfume down there before the appointment, and if that makes you feel more comfortable, then do it. But do it for yourself, because I know what to expect when I put my head down there and go to work. I know, and any professional in my field knows, what to expect, that there might be a faint smell of human but nothing that is bad. Never! If by some possibility, you know you have a infection of some sort, it is probably not a good idea to get a Brazilian wax during that time anyways, so reschedule your appointment if you suspect anything unusual going on with yourself. Otherwise, do not let the fear of smelling bad or of upsetting your esthetician with your smell, prevent from you coming in to get your wax job.

Pregnant

I love waxing pregnant women! It has been one of my most enlightening and educational experiences with women's bodies. I feel honored that I have had the opportunity to wax many guests for years before pregnancy, through pregnancy, and for years after.

> I have been getting Brazilians from Molly for many years. She is the best! I have two children now, and Molly waxed me before and through both my entire pregnancies. Although it does hurt a little more during pregnancy, it was well worth the pain. I felt clean and sexy, which can sometimes be hard while you're pregnant. Both times, we scheduled the waxes so that I would

get my last one right before delivery. I was able to feel fresh for weeks after the delivery. I appreciated her kind and professional approach toward this special time of my life and shared many conversations about how, as women, we should feel the most sexy during pregnancy. Thank you so much for your love, compassion, and determination to make all women feel like goddesses!

Lisa, 40, MD

It is totally safe to get waxed while you're pregnant. There are no contraindications for waxing during this time. However, the sensitivity will be similar to that of while you're menstruating. I usually suggest that my pregnant guests come every four weeks, to avoid any extra discomfort during this precious time.

Everything changes when you are pregnant. Your hormones are on overdrive during this time, so I'm never sure what to expect each month when I see you. Sometimes the hair goes into a rapid growth cycle, and for others, it slows way down. But it is an excellent time to continue getting your waxing done or even to receive your first wax.

I have only had two Brazilians in my life, and both have been done by Molly. I first did it as a surprise for my husband, just as a little turn-on. Then, I started doing it for me. I like the look and the feel of my skin after having a Brazilian done, and I also get a sense of empowerment, because I control how much hair is there and how much is not. The surprising thing for me is that I could handle having all that hair ripped out while being pregnant. I got the first one done at three months and the second at six months. I fully intend on keeping them up as long as my body can handle it. Molly knows exactly how to make me comfortable even when there is slight pain. She encourages breathing techniques, pillows for positioning, and anything else to make me feel comfortable. Molly is so well informed on Brazilian preparation, waxing techniques, and aftercare. She truly is a professional, and I love going to her. She is simply amazing.

Cassandra, 26, registered nurse/pregnant

Waxing helps many women continue to feel sexy during a time when not everyone feels so hot, even though—I'm sure you know what I'm going to say—I think all pregnant women should feel their absolute goddess selves during this honored time. The feedback I have gotten is that waxing helps pregnant women feel cleaner, as hormones usually cause that area to thrive with a juicier texture than usual.

I remember the first pregnant guest I had the opportunity to see through her entire pregnancy. I had been waxing her for years, and she came in one day with the good news that she was pregnant. Over the first few months, neither of us noticed any changes in her normal experience, pain-wise or anything else. Around the fifth month, she started really showing, with the beautiful bump that pops out on the belly. But we also noticed around this time that she was starting to get really sensitive to the wax job, emotionally and physically. So we went a little slower and really took our time. About the sixth month, I got down there to go to work, and I noticed that her vagina was changing. It had swelled a little, and the color was darker, with more blood and pressure in those vessels. By month seven and eight, I had to ask her when the last time was that she had really looked down there! It was like a whole new vagina. It was a shock to me too. I knew and had heard people lightly talk about the changes that happen, but I was looking right at it! It was full, radiant, and beautiful. She said that her husband had mentioned that it looked a little different, but that she had not really looked. I waxed her as kindly as I possibly could and made her look at her gorgeous self; it was emotional. She scheduled her last wax the same week she was due, so she could be clean for the delivery and the weeks after. Today, I have waxed hundreds of pregnant women through the entire term, and it is pretty much the same story with all my incredible baby-growing goddesses. We share this gifted time together. I love what I do.

After Babies and Hemorrhoids

I sometimes don't see a new mom for a couple months, but this is usually because she is at home, busy enjoying her new little bundle of joy. However, most of my new mommies want to stay on track with their Brazilians and continue coming a few weeks after delivery. The vagina is such an amazing thing. I won't go off on one of my beautiful vagina tangents, but it really is outstanding, what the female body is capable of … having babies! But I will admit that almost all women do look a little different after having children. In this paragraph, I want to discuss the time right after having a baby and all those moms who have children of many ages and their concerns. Right after having a baby, the area can be a little sore and still swollen for a couple months. This is still a safe and good time to continue receiving waxing. We will just go slowly and take the same extra precautions as when you were pregnant. With my moms who have had babies, whether it was one year ago or twenty, there still seems to be the same concerns and also some special cases. The number one concern, although they can happen to anyone, not just women who have delivered a baby … are hemorrhoids. Almost every woman who has had a baby has them. And every time, almost every woman who has one feels that she must warn me that it's ugly down there and that she must prepare me for what I'm about to see! Ladies, honestly, it's not as crazy-looking as you think, and most of my guests have them. Hemorrhoids do not scare me, and they certainly don't make you look ugly or disfigured down there! It is very easy to wax around them, and your esthetician will take the appropriate actions to avoid creating any discomfort. Some of my guests have given me feedback that removing the hair in the perianal area has relieved some of the discomfort associated with the hemorrhoids. I really believe that, in most of my guests' eyes, their tiny little normal hemorrhoid is this giant, huge thing that they believe is much larger than it really is. It is normal to have them, and you do not need to warn your esthetician that you have one or feel insecure about having them. I'm sure you're the tenth person with hemorrhoids they have seen in just that day alone. No big deal, I promise. This is another one of those goddess moments when I have had the opportunity, on several occasions, to let a woman know that she is still beautiful and sexy down there.

I had one guest in particular, a mom of three in her forties, who didn't even start to undress until she fully described what I was going to see once she took her underwear off. I assured her that I had seen many hemorrhoids before and that she would be fine. After the wax, she admitted to me that she hasn't let husband look at her in the light for several years and has not let him explore her body down there too much in those years either. She came back the next month with a different story! She thanked me and told me that having another person look at her spread open with everything revealed, and being told by someone who sees naked women all day that she looked absolutely normal and beautiful, helped her tremendously with her healing. She also described how having that experience with me, along with her new Brazilian, ignited her relationship with her husband, and things were going better than ever in and out of the bedroom. Her newfound confidence made her feel sexy and relaxed, so she could truly enjoy her husband again. I love my job!

Now that the big concern of hemorrhoids is out of the way, I should mention some special cases. Some women, during delivery, can experience some damage to their vaginas. I have seen one side of the labia to be stretched and uneven from the other side, or one labia may be permanently swollen with broken blood vessels. Again, this is all normal, and we are accustomed to seeing these sorts of after-babies results. To be honest, I have even seen this in women who have not had babies, so please don't feel you are damaged or changed since having children. Yes, it happens mostly to women who have delivered babies, but it can also be natural. So, whether you are a veteran waxer who is wondering if you should continue after babies, or you are considering your first wax, know that your esthetician is prepared to give you a Brazilian and remind you of the sexy woman you are!

Different Shapes and Sizes

I'm not going to say that we are all snowflakes, and no two look alike. I would say ... there are a couple of molds from which we all came from, and then we each have some unique flair that sets us apart. It breaks my heart, as I mentioned before, that almost every single woman apologizes for something about her vagina before she undresses. One of these apologies is preparing me for how it's going to look down there. Sometimes the apology is that it's crazy overgrown with hair ... I know, that's why you're here! Then there are those moments when they let me know they have an extremely pronounced labia or clit or that the whole thing is huge. They are all beautiful ... and I will admit that, in my younger days, when I would look at naked photos of women and would see women with these glorious giant, full, and huge vaginas, I would get jealous. I suppose, like penis envy, I had vagina envy! They are all beautiful. I have witnessed many of these women, whether they are small or giant, experience a healing once they have decided to start Brazilians—a testament to themselves that, here it is, big or small, I love it and am choosing to acknowledge its existence! They are all beautiful …

The best moments are watching those ladies who don't even know what they have going on down there. This might sound corny, but it's totally honest. A woman will come in for her first Brazilian, and maybe she is just getting it for a vacation, so that no pubes will show out of her suit. Or, for example, I have several guests who are champion horse riders, and they decide to get a Brazilian to avoid the irritation they experience from the hours they spend in the saddle. But they have never really looked at it. Although every woman is a new experience for me, to watch these ladies' expressions is amazing. As I begin to remove the wrapping paper of hair to reveal the hidden gift inside, I never know which kind of snowflake I will find. But when the entire veil of hair is gone, and it's time to look at yourself … some women just stare at it. They have never really looked at every fold, crease, color, and opening.… They have never looked at their true source of power. They have never looked at why all men just think about sex every day. They have never looked at why we are so magnificent, and why this hidden spot is the creation of all life. It brings babies into the world! It brings joy to the world! You and your vagina's are all beautiful, mysterious, and perfect. I love these moments.

There is no way of predicting what I'm going to see, by a person's outer appearance. I had better address some of these myths. The tiniest, most petite woman can come in, who has never had children, and she might have a very pronounced vagina. A very largely built woman can come in, who has had four babies and loves lots of sex, and she might have the smallest vagina. I have had many virgins come in to get waxed for their wedding night, and some of these ladies have pronounced, fleshy, and huge vaginas. I have seen porn videos and heard men talk about how huge some women's vaginas are, but I have to say, being of some vagina expertise, that the regular virgin might have one of these too. Babies might stretch you out a *little*, seriously, just a little, and maybe change your appearance, but I have seen the same thing on an eighteen-year-old virgin. And you know what? I have had many conversations with men for research and curiosity, and they love them all. Some men even have preferences for a nice, little innie or for a full, huge outie! They are all beautiful.

So, please do not avoid a Brazilian wax because of some fear of your size, shape, or even of seeing it in its totally hairless beauty. Let's not hide it anymore—set it free!

Sex and Anal Sex

I'm sure you can only imagine the kind of conversations I have inside my little room! I decided to include this little mention, since it seems to come up on a weekly basis. Everyone wants to know if I can tell if she had sex the night before or if she had anal sex. No, ladies, I can't. I had one client, who had come to me for years, apologize before her appointment that it might look crazy down there since her husband, who I know and is sweet and loving, had had tequila the night before and had gotten wild. I laughed, and I really looked—the ever-wondering student in me—but could not see any difference in her vagina from the usual. So, go ahead and have wild sex the night before your appointment; no one will ever know!

I have had several situations where one of my usual clients has had anal sex recently and is concerned that I can tell or that the perianal area will be too sensitive to wax. Okay, so I can't tell if you had anal sex the night before, but I will be honest and say that this area is extra-sensitive in my guests who participate in this activity. If it's extremely swollen or sore, I will avoid waxing the perianal area that day. But usually, if I pretreat the area with a little extra oil before I lay down the wax, then everything will go well. We are always a team during waxing, so if it hurts, we stop. Work with your esthetician, and always be honest, so your treatment and experience go as smoothly as possible.

Do Men Get Waxed Down There?

Of course! Some men love being totally clean and hairless, just like women. Today, the idea of metrosexual is common knowledge. There are a few special cares, however, in doing a man's wax. The scrotum can not be waxed. The skin is so thin on this fragile part of a man, that no esthetician should ever try it. The skin will come right off, and you will have an emergency on your hands. But the pubic hair surrounding the shaft and penis is very safe to have waxed. To be honest, most men do not keep up with that part of the wax. Most of my male guests are all big fans of having their butt cracks waxed. They might try the whole thing, front to back, several times, but most will only continue with the perianal wax on a regular basis and keep themselves groomed in the front area at home, with clippers or scissors. The feedback I get from my men is similar to my female guests' feedback. They love feeling clean, especially in their butt cracks! The funny thing they always tell me that is graphic but good information—they don't need to use as much toilet paper!

So, if your husband or boyfriend has ever complained of feeling sweaty or too hairy down there, ask your esthetician if she is comfortable with performing male Brazilians. An experienced and professional waxer will have no problem with this and will guide them through the experience.

Can I Wax Myself?

Okay, so this isn't really an embarrassing question, but it's definitely a question I get asked often. It is also one of those questions that people are nervous to ask, since they want an honest answer but don't want me to feel like I might lose their business.

I know of several women who are able to wax themselves, but they have been doing it for years and do it often, like twice a month. Or it also works if you have been getting waxes done by a professional for years, and you hardly grow hair anymore, so doing it at home is much easier. This is not easy, ladies, coming from my own experience! As I explained in an earlier chapter, I have gone to every Brazilian waxer out there, because I wanted to learn from their art, and I love and adore having a wax myself. I have yet to find someone as thorough as myself, so I have tried twice to do myself. Oh, man, just thinking about those incidents now makes my skin crawl! Let me say first, that I wax everything else myself—my legs, brows, arms, and upper lip. The other thing I can't do myself is my underarms … a discussion for another time. It is extremely difficult to go so far outside of your head to inflict that kind of pain on yourself and yet be alert enough to do the pull properly. Although I have done yoga for years, I would need to be extremely flexible to contort myself enough to lay the wax properly! So, the first time I tried to give myself a Brazilian, I was home alone with a mirror propped up on the bathroom floor, spread wide open with everything ready to go. I laid the wax down on my lip area, pressed the cloth onto myself, gave myself a pep talk, and pulled! Wowzers! I bruised myself so badly that it felt like I had pulled my insides out. As I mentioned earlier, if you pull straight up from the body, it will cause you to bruise. Well, I'm an esthetician, not a circus performer, so no matter how I tried, I could not do the proper pull when working on myself. So, now I'm stuck with wax in my inner lips and butt crack and panicking! I grabbed a bottle of olive oil and poured it everywhere … oil eats oil, just like you use peanut butter to get gum out of hair. After an hour of massaging olive oil and dissolving the wax, I finally was free of this nightmare.

Ever the believer in myself, I tried it once more a few months later. This time, my boyfriend was home, so I recruited him to help. I let him practice a few pulls on my leg first to get the idea of how much of an art goes into the perfect pull. He wasn't great but good enough. I laid the wax on my lips, pressed the cloth, and held my own skin tightly. Once it was pull time, he got really nervous and started giving himself a pep talk! Finally, we took a deep breath, and he pulled. It was worse than if I had done it myself … let's just say I started bleeding, and he fainted! Once he came to, which was pretty quickly, he was pail and terrified! We got the olive oil, and massaged the remainder of wax off my area, so we could see what was going on down there. He had pulled so fast and aggressively that it had torn my inner labia just a tiny bit. No big deal, but it scared the heck out of both of us! I healed within a few days but have never done myself again.

I will also mention that women come in with similar stories on a daily basis. They have tried waxing at home several times with disastrous outcomes of every nature. I also have those select women who have done themselves for years, who love the luxury of coming in once in a while to avoid the mind over pain that month and to ensure a perfectly clean wax job. So what do I suggest here? If you really want to try doing it yourself, work your way up to it *slowly* and maybe do a few strips every week, working your way into the inner lips. But success with this is so rare that, of course, I recommend just going to a professional and getting it done right! You deserve this gift to yourself. It's worth the cost for the extra attention and perfection.

Chapter 10
Testimonials

Just in case you're still not convinced that you should take the hairless challenge, I have decided to include more testimonials! I have been overwhelmed by the responses I have received from my guests. As I began receiving and reading them, I experienced every emotion possible. Some made me cry, some made me laugh, and some made me feel immense gratitude! These guests are my harem, my joy, and my inspiration for my own journey of healing. But most of all, I feel a deep, soulful thankfulness. Thank you…. I love what I do…. Thank you, universe… Thank you, Divine Feminine…. Thank you, harem…. Thank you, sisters…. Thank you…. Because of you *women*, I am so blessed, grateful, and passionate about what I do. I love what I do, because of you…. Thank you …

> I have been married for twelve years. My husband and I have a great sex life, and we are always interested in trying new things. One of his requests was for me to shave. I hated it. Standing in the shower with one leg propped up on the shower wall, or practically on my head, trying to reach all the appropriate areas, then little bumps, a couple days and, shazam, it would all be back again like some small creature had overtaken. I did it only because he really liked it; but thank *God* birthdays and anniversaries only came once a year.

> One year, I decided to get waxed. What the heck. It couldn't be any more obnoxious than what I'd been through previously, and I heard it lasted much longer. I made an appointment and was given a list of choices. I chose the full Brazilian. I figured,

what the heck, if I was going to do it, I might as well *really* do it. So, although I still managed to have my legs up in the air in full yoga fashion, the whole thing was done in twenty minutes! And, yes, it hurt. It didn't hurt like an appendicitis or childbirth. It hurt like a slap or a Band-Aid, which actually is about what it was like. The pain was over before I got dressed.

I felt lighter. Don't ask me why; it's not like she took off three pounds of hair (thank God). I also felt naughty. I didn't look any different. I wore the same clothes I came with, and I didn't walk differently or learn to speak another language.

That night, I made supper (probably something boring like meat loaf) but couldn't stop smiling. My husband had no idea what was about to happen. No anniversary, no birthday, probably a Tuesday ... cleaned the kitchen, put the kids to bed, read stories, and, yes, I'm dragging this out.

Without getting super graphic here, my husband freaked out. He "freaked out" a couple times that night, met me for lunch, and "freaked out" a couple times again the next night. I have no idea why; it was just naughty. No new moves, no new positions. I will admit to oral sex, though. He said there was no hair to tickle his nose. It became a secret between us. Who knows why it excited him so much, but I'll tell you that the added attention and his great reaction from it was worth every minute of the waxing procedure. And it was smooth for *weeks*! No bumps, no rash, no scratchy regrowth. I even got a promotion at work! Just kidding.

Pam, 34, mother of two/housewife

I first decided to get a Brazilian wax about two-and-a-half years ago and haven't looked back since. It was just by chance that I booked my first wax with Molly, but after that first time, I couldn't possibly go to anyone else. Her skill and expertise is apparent after your first visit. She has the best kind of personality that you immediately can connect with. She is a kind and loving soul; both of these aspects shine through her work. Not only are the results good for your physical physique but also for you spiritually. For whatever reason, in our fifteen-minute sessions, we would have the deepest conversations about everything; she is my wax therapist. I could go on forever singing her praise. I highly recommend Molly and have, to many friends.

Zoë, 24, student

My husband at the time pressured me into getting my first Brazilian wax. I went the first time for him, but we are no longer together, and I continue to go as a single woman. They are for me and only me. I love feeling smooth and sexy. I love looking at myself that way and feeling myself that way. It is part of my lifestyle and forever will be.

Heather, 45, single/parole officer

I decided to get a Brazilian on a suggestion (to put it mildly) from my husband. I am in my fifties, and my husband and I have been together for twenty-two years. We have always enjoyed an intimate relationship, and I have always considered myself to be open-minded.

I thought I was getting the Brazilian for my husband. I knew he would be very pleased with the result (and he has been!), but I didn't anticipate that it would also be stimulating for me. His enthusiasm has been infectious. He is so excited every time I go in for a waxing. He is like a kid in a candy store.

Who would have thought that a simple thing could give so much pleasure?

Jana, 50-something, government employee

I have been getting Brazilian waxes since I was a junior in college. I always had problems with shaving, because my skin was just too sensitive. Since that first wax, I have not had one problem, and I was completely addicted! It's absolutely the best thing I have ever decided to do! It started as a surprise for my boyfriend (now husband), who lived in Colorado while I was living in Texas, going to school. He was addicted from the first time too! To this day, he gets so excited on the days I get a wax! Not only does it make me feel feminine and sexy, but it also makes me feel clean! It's something that I get to do for myself to make me feel better, and my husband just happens to enjoy it as well! I couldn't imagine not having it done on a regular basis, and now that I've found the absolute best person to do it ... I wouldn't trade it for the world! When I moved to Colorado, I found Molly by chance and now have several people from work going to her regularly and loving it too! I would recommend this to anyone!

Ashley, 25, nurse

Finding a high-quality sexual partner (for the first time) after age fifty was a complete surprise to me. Keeping my man happy keeps me happy. Brazilian waxing is the only way to fly. Yahoo!

BeeDo, 59, appraiser

Her boyfriend commented:

Banana-smoothies are the rage today!

Happy contractor, 63

I am not what you would call an adventurous sort; in fact, I am quite modest but also a self-confident woman who doesn't wear an ounce of makeup. But, I decided that I needed to get a bikini wax to get things under control. I proceeded cautiously; interviewing friends about just how invasive this bikini waxing was ... would I have to get naked? Am I too, well, not size 4? Will I die of embarrassment? The answers were mixed, but I decided to go for it. However, it was not until I met my present esthetician, Molly, that I was going for the gusto ... she easily talked me into a Brazilian and, well, I never went back!

The truth is, it really hurts so good! It makes me happy, simple as that, and my partner enjoys it as well! I must admit I am addicted!

Thanks for that!

Lynn F., 33, wildlife ecologist

A Brazilian wax? Are you kidding? Well ... Molly eased me into one with her usual grace, intuition, expertise, and healing ways. Frankly, I didn't even know Brazil was on my horizon. Thank you, Molly, for being in my life and for helping me discover my inner goddess.

Sam, 60, retiree

In Conclusion
One More Thing, Just for Fun!

Just for fun, I thought I would write down every word I have ever heard for our vaginas! I asked everyone I knew, including men. I understand there are different levels of understanding for some of these ... we consider some as degrading. However, this is just for fun so please laugh or even use one you have never heard of someday, but please do not be offended.

Honey hole	Bear trap	Hooha
Pie hole	Dew flaps	Jade gate
Love nest	Downstairs	Sugar basin
Cunt	Moneymaker	Vertical smile
Twat	Mouth that can't bite	Upright wink
Slit	Fanny	Undercarriage
Pink taco	Nether regions	Cock holster
Love tunnel	Delta of Venus	Beefgina
Victory hole	Beef curtains	Wee-wee
Juice box	Oracle	Vage
Love canal	Flesh tuxedo	Home
	(from the movie *This Is Spinal Tap*)	
Coochie	Bermuda triangle	Love glove
Africa	Coozie	Crotch
Pussy	Flower	Snatch

Hair pie	Pink velvet sausage wallet	Sword sheath
Fur burger	Front bum	Vajeen (from *Borat*)
Peach	Joy box	Penis fly trap
Vajajay	IT	Cookie
Meat drapes	Man in the boat (clitoris)	Kitty
Carpet	Cooter	Muffin
Muff	Front parlor	Cum dumpster
Poonani	Madge	Axe wound
Landing strip	Vaj	Fun hole
Beaver	Gash	Vaginator
Tuna	Bush	Trouser tarantula
Rug	Garden of Eden	The show
Glory hole	Bikini triangle	Yammer
Cherry pie	Cave	Stinky pinky
The Y	Pootang	Hot pocket
Camel toe	Pleasure garden	Bean pod
Ace of spades	Loins	The lovin' oven
Queen of hearts	Yoni	Fortune cookie
Afro clam	Rosebud	Hot dog bun
Bearded clam	Bread box	Flapjack
Altar of love	Heaven's door	Hanging hamburger
Baby cave	Pooter	Landing gear
Attic	Jam cookie	Junk
Badger	Booty	Hairy yo-yo
Mossy cottage	Silent beard	Winker

I have to address this page of fun names.... I could not believe what kind of a reaction it stirred! I only knew a few of the names myself, and then I had to break out and start asking other circles. Men had the worst ones and some of the sweetest ones (my personal favorite came from someone I admire: honey hole!). Worst only in terms of being incredibly graphic, I didn't even want to write some of them down, and there is no one more open than I! I would be at a dinner party asking some of the men what they have heard vaginas called, and it would start the most incredible conversations. I couldn't believe the stories surrounding why they came up with that name, or maybe their older brother told them that's what vaginas were called when they were kids. In some instances, it made me feel sad, because, as young boys, they should have only grown up thinking of the vagina as beautiful and magnificent ... not as a "cum dumpster." I will accept the word cunt as maybe erotic and sexy at times, but axe wound? I have a sick sense of humor, so I can see where some of the names are funny but disgusting. However, I can see where children hearing these names might begin to think of the vagina as something that is gross or as something not to be appreciated for its own perfection. Here goes my goddess talk again.... We have to, as women, and men are just as responsible, to raise our children with the knowledge of how sacred and amazing our bodies are! That begins with us. We have to start acknowledging our perfection, beauty, and magnificence. Today, right now, we must find a way to see ourselves as goddesses!

I believe and hope that a Brazilian wax is one of those ways to guide you to seeing your true self. Then, hopefully we can raise our children to appreciate themselves.... I believe this goes as far as teaching good health for our vaginas. Beyond the recognition and appreciation of our vaginas, comes the most important lesson—the health of our vaginas. If we begin to see them for how great they are, then we will begin to take better care of them on every level. This will transcend into teaching our daughters to love, admire, and respect their vaginas! So important, so vital, so necessary ... I could have used this perspective when I was young.

On the flip side of coin, I work with over fifty women in my salon and spa, so I decided to put up a huge piece of paper in the break room stating for everyone to write down every name they have ever heard. This was amazing.... The first few hours, I noticed that no one wrote anything down. I asked a couple girls what was up ... and I was told that a few of the women were offended by my poster—which is exactly why we need to talk about this! So I approached the few women. They told me if it was just for fun, it seemed offensive, but if it had a purpose that would be different. So I had to let the cat out of the bag ... I had been working on this opus for over a year and had not told anyone about it. So I told the staff what I was up to, and the reaction was overwhelming! Everyone was so excited and suddenly couldn't wait to share their stories with me. It was beautiful! After hearing the men's response, it was interesting to watch the women. There were certainly a few stories that pissed me off, of how women had felt demoralized about their sacred spot from when they were just young girls. But mostly it started vagina conversation of the best kind! Once the seal was broken, stories and discussion started flowing. These women couldn't wait to tell their messages. The most interesting angle for me was hearing what their children had named their own privates! Those are on the list too ... and they are just as important, because these kids formed their own names for how they associated the vagina in connection with themselves and the world—beautiful! I heard what Grandma called it and the great story behind it. It made me realize how connected we all are about something so huge, yet everyone is nervous to talk about it. My grandma, mother, and sisters, each in their own way taught me about my vagina and my sexuality, through how they perceived their own. My grandma, although a feminist, made me think it was dirty all the time. My mother, taught me the importance of keeping it healthy and sacred. My sisters and my cousin taught me how to enjoy it.

We all have these stories that have formed our recognition of our vaginas, which in turn have affected how we see ourselves as women. How we view our vaginas is how we view our worth in many ways. It affects our sexuality, intimacy, relationships, and self-esteem. Today, begin to see yourself through your vagina ... its experiences, what it has been told it is, and how it has reacted. I know this may seem silly, but seriously think about it for a moment—if we really could accept the truth of our perfection through our vaginas and their very purpose to bring life and joy. Maybe then we can begin to see ourselves as entire human beings who deserve life, joy, and happiness. Let's be good to our vaginas. Let's begin to teach our children of their worth and beauty. Let's begin to nurture ourselves so that everyone around us will begin to nurture one another. Global vagina love!